Table of Contents

INTRODUCTION...3

UNDERSTANDING YOUR VAGUS NERVE 7

THE VAGUS NERVE DIET..11

    UNDERSTANDING THE VAGUS NERVE DIET:............11

    MINDFUL EATING PRACTICES 14

    STRESS REDUCTION TECHNIQUES............................18

    HOLISTIC HEALING: NURTURING MIND, BODY, AND SPIRIT 22

VAGUS NERVE DIET COOKBOOK 27

    BREAKFAST..27

    LUNCH 43

    DINNER..60

    SNACKS...83

    DESSERTS 93

CONCLUSION...105

INTRODUCTION

I welcome you to the world of culinary wellness, where the flavors of food meet the science of well-being! In this cookbook, I embark on a delightful journey into the realm of the vagus nerve, a remarkable part of our nervous system that plays a pivotal role in our overall health and happiness. "Nourish Your Nerve: A Cookbook for Living Well with the Vagus Nerve" is your comprehensive guide to understanding and nourishing this essential nerve, allowing you to unlock the full potential of your mind-body connection and experience a life of vitality and balance.

The vagus nerve, often referred to as the "wandering nerve," is a complex and dynamic neural highway that connects your brain to various vital organs throughout your body, including your heart, lungs, digestive system, and more. This remarkable nerve regulates a wide range of essential functions, such as heart rate, digestion, inflammation, and even emotional well-being. It's the key to your body's ability to rest and digest, to heal, and to thrive.

In recent years, scientific research has revealed the profound influence of the vagus nerve on our physical and mental health. It's now understood that the health of this nerve is closely linked to conditions like anxiety, depression, chronic inflammation, and digestive disorders. Furthermore, it plays a pivotal role in our body's relaxation response, helping us manage stress and maintain a state of balance and harmony.

This cookbook is your passport to a more vibrant and fulfilling life by nourishing and nurturing your vagus nerve through the power of food. Each recipe is carefully crafted to support and enhance the health of your vagus nerve, promoting better digestion, reduced inflammation, improved mental clarity, and emotional well-being. From savory soups to indulgent desserts, every dish is a celebration of flavors and well-being.

Inside "Nourish Your Nerve," you'll find:

• Understanding Your Vagus Nerve: I'll dive deep into the science behind the vagus nerve, explaining how it works and why it's crucial for your overall health.

• The Vagus Nerve Diet: Discover the foods that are known to stimulate and support the vagus nerve, helping you create a balanced and nourishing meal plan.

• Recipes for Wellness: My collection of delicious recipes spans breakfast, lunch, dinner, snacks, and desserts, all designed to provide the nutrients and flavors that your vagus nerve craves.

• Mindful Eating Practices: Learn how to incorporate mindfulness into your meals, allowing you to fully savor each bite and reap the benefits of conscious eating.

• Stress Reduction Techniques: Explore simple yet effective techniques to reduce stress and enhance your vagal tone, such as deep breathing exercises, meditation, and yoga.

• Holistic Healing: Discover other complementary practices, such as herbal remedies and aromatherapy, that can further support your vagus nerve health.

Are you ready to embark on a journey toward a healthier, happier you? "Nourish Your Nerve" is your guide to living well by nourishing your vagus nerve through the joy of cooking and mindful eating. As you explore these pages and savor the delectable recipes within, may you find not only satisfaction for your taste buds but also a path to enhanced well-being and a more harmonious life. Let's embark on this delicious voyage together!

UNDERSTANDING YOUR VAGUS NERVE

The vagus nerve, also known as the cranial nerve X, is a remarkable and intricate part of the autonomic nervous system. It is the longest of the cranial nerves, extending from the brainstem through the neck and into the chest and abdomen. The word "vagus" itself is derived from the Latin word for "wandering," aptly describing the nerve's meandering path throughout the body.

This nerve is a two-way communication superhighway that carries information between your brain and various organs and systems throughout your body. Its primary function is to regulate and maintain balance in many essential bodily functions, both consciously and unconsciously. Here are some key aspects to understanding the vagus nerve:

• Parasympathetic Nervous System: The vagus nerve is a crucial component of the parasympathetic nervous system, often referred to as the "rest and digest" or "feed and breed" system. When activated, it helps the body relax, slow down, and conserve energy. This activation is essential for processes like digestion, reducing heart rate, and promoting calmness.

• Brain-Gut Connection: The vagus nerve plays a pivotal role in the gut-brain connection. It carries signals from the digestive system to the brain and vice versa. This bi-directional communication influences emotions, mood, and even mental health. A healthy vagus nerve can contribute to better emotional regulation and resilience.

• Heart Health: The vagus nerve helps regulate heart rate and rhythm. When the vagus nerve is stimulated, it slows down the heart rate, contributing to cardiovascular stability. An active vagus nerve is associated with lower heart disease risk.

• Inflammation Control: This nerve also plays a role in regulating inflammation throughout the body.

Vagus nerve activation can help reduce inflammatory responses, which are implicated in various chronic diseases.

• Respiratory Function: It influences breathing patterns and respiratory rate. Deep, slow breathing can stimulate the vagus nerve and promote relaxation.

• Social Engagement: The vagus nerve is involved in social interactions and facial expressions. It plays a role in connecting with others, empathy, and bonding.

• Stress Response: A healthy vagus nerve can help modulate the body's stress response, making it easier to recover from stressful situations.

• Digestion: It controls the muscles that contract in the digestive tract, aiding in digestion and nutrient absorption. An active vagus nerve promotes healthy digestion and can help alleviate digestive disorders.

• Voice and Speech: The vagus nerve also influences the muscles involved in speech and vocalization.

Understanding your vagus nerve and its functions is essential for promoting overall well-being. The health of this nerve can be influenced by lifestyle factors such as diet, exercise, stress management, and mindful practices like meditation and deep breathing. By nourishing and stimulating your vagus nerve, you can enhance your body's ability to maintain balance, reduce stress, and support various aspects of physical and mental health.

THE VAGUS NERVE DIET

The Vagus Nerve Diet is a dietary approach aimed at supporting and enhancing the health of the vagus nerve, a crucial component of the autonomic nervous system. This diet focuses on incorporating foods and nutrients that promote vagus nerve function, leading to improved overall well-being, reduced stress, better digestion, and enhanced emotional resilience.

UNDERSTANDING THE VAGUS NERVE DIET:

• Anti-Inflammatory Foods: Chronic inflammation can impair vagus nerve function. The Vagus Nerve Diet emphasizes anti-inflammatory foods such as fatty fish (e.g., salmon, mackerel), leafy greens, berries, turmeric, ginger, and nuts. These foods help reduce inflammation and support vagus nerve health.

• Fiber-Rich Foods: A healthy gut is essential for vagus nerve function, and fiber-rich foods like whole grains, legumes, fruits, and vegetables promote gut health. They also aid in digestion and provide a source of nourishment for beneficial gut bacteria.

• Probiotics and Fermented Foods: Incorporating probiotics and fermented foods such as yogurt, kefir, sauerkraut, and kimchi can help maintain a balanced gut microbiome. A healthy gut contributes to improved vagus nerve signaling and emotional well-being.

• Omega-3 Fatty Acids: Foods rich in omega-3 fatty acids, like fatty fish, flaxseeds, and walnuts, support heart health and can help reduce inflammation, indirectly benefiting the vagus nerve.

• Leafy Greens and Vegetables: Leafy greens and vegetables are packed with vitamins, minerals, and antioxidants that promote overall health. They also contain fiber, which supports gut health.

• Herbs and Spices: Turmeric, ginger, and garlic are known for their anti-inflammatory properties and can be incorporated into dishes to enhance flavor and health benefits.

• Healthy Fats: Incorporate healthy fats from sources such as avocados, olive oil, and nuts. These fats support brain health and may aid in vagus nerve function.

• Limit Sugar and Processed Foods: High sugar and processed foods can contribute to inflammation and negatively impact gut health. Reducing or eliminating these from your diet can support vagus nerve health.

• Hydration: Staying well-hydrated is essential for overall health. Water supports various bodily functions, including digestion and circulation, which can indirectly influence the vagus nerve.

• Mindful Eating: Eating mindfully, slowly, and without distractions can enhance digestion and activate the vagus nerve's rest and digest response. Engaging in mindful eating practices can be as important as the foods you consume.

It's important to note that individual dietary needs may vary. Before making significant changes to your diet, consult with a healthcare professional or registered dietitian, especially if you have specific medical conditions or dietary restrictions.

Incorporating the Vagus Nerve Diet into your lifestyle can be a holistic approach to improving overall health and well-being. By nourishing your vagus nerve with nutrient-rich foods and adopting mindful eating practices, you can take an active role in promoting balance, reducing stress, and enhancing your body's natural ability to heal and thrive.

MINDFUL EATING PRACTICES

Mindful eating is a practice that encourages a deep awareness of your eating habits, sensations, thoughts, and emotions related to food. It promotes a more conscious and intentional approach to eating, fostering a healthier relationship with food, and supporting overall well-being. Here are some mindful eating practices to help you develop a more mindful approach to your meals:

• Savor Each Bite: Take the time to truly savor and appreciate the flavors, textures, and aromas of your food. Pay attention to the different tastes on your palate and how they change as you chew.

• Eat Without Distractions: Minimize distractions while eating. Turn off the TV, put away your smartphone, and create a peaceful environment at the dining table. This allows you to focus solely on your meal.

• Use All Your Senses: Engage all your senses in the eating experience. Notice the colors, shapes, and presentation of your food. Listen to the sounds it makes as you eat. Touch your food and appreciate its texture.

• Chew Thoroughly: Take the time to chew your food slowly and thoroughly. Chewing aids digestion and allows you to connect more deeply with the sensory experience of eating.

• Appreciate Your Food's Journey: Consider the journey your food has taken from farm to table. Reflect on the effort and resources that went into producing, preparing, and serving your meal. This can increase gratitude and awareness.

• Recognize Hunger and Fullness: Pay attention to your body's hunger and fullness cues. Eat when you are genuinely hungry, and stop when you are comfortably satisfied. Avoid eating out of boredom or emotional triggers.

• Mindful Portion Control: Be mindful of portion sizes. Serve yourself smaller portions and give yourself the option to have seconds if you are still hungry. This can help prevent overeating.

• Slow Down: Eating slowly not only aids digestion but also allows your brain to catch up with your stomach's fullness signals. Put your utensils down between bites to pace yourself.

• Practice Gratitude: Before you begin your meal, take a moment to express gratitude for the food in front of you and for the nourishment it provides. This can foster a more positive relationship with food.

• Engage in Conversation: If you are dining with others, engage in meaningful conversation. Sharing meals and connecting with loved ones can enhance the enjoyment of your food.

• Take Breaks: If you're having a multi-course meal, take short breaks between courses to check in with your body's hunger and fullness cues.

• Be Nonjudgmental: Approach your eating experience with kindness and self-compassion. If you find yourself veering off the mindful path, acknowledge it without judgment and gently guide yourself back to the present moment.

• Reflect on Food Choices: After your meal, reflect on the choices you made and how your body feels.

This reflection can help you become more attuned to your body's needs and preferences.

STRESS REDUCTION TECHNIQUES

In my fast-paced and demanding world, stress is an almost inevitable part of life. However, managing and reducing stress is crucial for our mental and physical well-being. Here are some effective stress reduction techniques that can help you find calm in the midst of chaos:

• Deep Breathing: Practicing deep, diaphragmatic breathing can quickly calm your nervous system. Try the 4-7-8 technique: Inhale for a count of 4, hold for a count of 7, and exhale for a count of 8. Repeat this several times.

• Mindfulness Meditation: Mindfulness meditation involves focusing your attention on the present moment without judgment. Regular practice can reduce stress and improve emotional regulation.

You can use guided meditation apps or simply focus on your breath and sensations.

• Progressive Muscle Relaxation: This technique involves tensing and then releasing each muscle group in your body, starting from your toes and moving up to your head. It helps relieve physical tension.

• Yoga: Yoga combines physical postures, breathing exercises, and meditation. It's an excellent way to reduce stress, improve flexibility, and promote relaxation.

• Tai Chi: Tai Chi is a slow and graceful form of exercise that combines movement, deep breathing, and meditation. It can help reduce stress, improve balance, and increase energy flow.

• Exercise: Regular physical activity releases endorphins, which are natural mood lifters. Find an activity you enjoy, whether it's walking, jogging, dancing, or swimming, and make it a part of your routine.

• Nature Walks: Spending time in nature has been shown to reduce stress and promote a sense of well-being. Take a walk in a park, forest, or any natural setting to connect with the outdoors.

• Journaling: Writing down your thoughts and feelings can help you process stressors and gain clarity. You can also use journaling to focus on gratitude and positive aspects of your life.

• Social Connection: Sharing your thoughts and concerns with a trusted friend or family member can provide emotional support and reduce feelings of isolation. Building and maintaining social connections is vital for stress management.

• Limit Screen Time: Excessive screen time, especially on social media and news websites, can increase stress and anxiety. Set boundaries for screen time and take regular breaks.

• Mindful Eating: Practice mindful eating (as mentioned earlier) to enjoy your food fully and reduce stress related to emotional or mindless eating.

• Aromatherapy: Certain scents, such as lavender, chamomile, and eucalyptus, can promote relaxation and reduce stress. Try using essential oils or scented candles in your daily routine.

• Art and Creative Expression: Engage in creative activities like drawing, painting, or crafting. These activities can be therapeutic and provide an outlet for stress.

• Music: Listen to calming music or sounds of nature to relax your mind and reduce stress. Consider creating a playlist of your favorite soothing tunes.

• Time Management: Organize your tasks and set realistic priorities. Avoid overloading your schedule, and take breaks to recharge during the day.

• Professional Help: If stress becomes overwhelming or persistent, consider seeking support from a mental health professional, such as a therapist or counselor.

HOLISTIC HEALING: NURTURING MIND, BODY, AND SPIRIT

Holistic healing is an approach to health and well-being that considers the whole person—mind, body, and spirit—rather than focusing solely on specific symptoms or diseases. It recognizes the interconnectedness of all aspects of an individual's life and seeks to promote balance and harmony in these areas. Holistic healing embraces a wide range of therapies and practices that aim to support natural healing processes and improve overall quality of life. Here are key components and approaches within holistic healing:

• Mind-Body Connection: Holistic healing recognizes the profound connection between the mind and the body. It emphasizes the impact of thoughts, emotions, and beliefs on physical health.

Practices like meditation, mindfulness, and visualization are used to harness the mind's power to influence well-being.

• Nutrition and Diet: Proper nutrition is essential for holistic health. A balanced diet rich in whole foods, fruits, vegetables, and nutrients can support physical well-being and boost the body's ability to heal itself. Some holistic approaches focus on specific diets tailored to individual needs.

• Exercise and Movement: Regular physical activity is crucial for overall health. Exercise not only strengthens the body but also helps release endorphins, which reduce stress and improve mood. Holistic healing often includes activities like yoga, Tai Chi, and Qi Gong for their physical and mental benefits.

• Alternative and Complementary Therapies: Holistic healing encompasses a wide range of therapies beyond conventional medicine. These may include acupuncture, chiropractic care, massage therapy, aromatherapy, herbal remedies, and energy healing practices like Reiki.

• Spirituality and Inner Balance: Nurturing the spirit is a vital component of holistic healing. This may involve connecting with one's inner self, practicing mindfulness or meditation, exploring one's beliefs, or engaging in spiritual practices that provide a sense of purpose and meaning.

• Stress Reduction: Stress is a significant contributor to many health issues. Holistic healing often includes stress-reduction techniques, such as mindfulness meditation, deep breathing exercises, and relaxation therapies, to promote emotional and physical well-being.

• Environmental Considerations: Holistic health takes into account the environment and its impact on health. This includes assessing the quality of air, water, and the living environment to reduce exposure to toxins and create a healthy living space.

- Emotional and Mental Health: Holistic healing recognizes the importance of emotional and mental health in overall well-being. Psychotherapy, counseling, and emotional support are valued components of holistic care.

- Individualized Care: Holistic healing is highly individualized. It recognizes that each person is unique and may require different approaches to healing. Practitioners often consider a person's physical, emotional, and spiritual needs when developing a treatment plan.

- Preventative Care: Holistic healing places a strong emphasis on preventative measures to maintain health and well-being. Regular health screenings, a healthy lifestyle, and early intervention are key aspects of holistic health care.

- Holistic Healthcare Practitioners: Holistic healing is often facilitated by practitioners who specialize in various holistic therapies, such as naturopathic doctors, holistic nurses, chiropractors, and herbalists.

Holistic healing does not necessarily replace conventional medical treatments but often complements them. It encourages individuals to take an active role in their health and well-being and to explore a wide range of approaches to support their holistic health journey. Ultimately, holistic healing seeks to empower individuals to achieve balance, vitality, and a sense of wholeness in their lives.

VAGUS NERVE DIET COOKBOOK

BREAKFAST

Avocado and Poached Egg Toast:

Ingredients:

- 1 slice of whole-grain bread

- 1/2 ripe avocado, mashed

- 1 poached egg

- Salt and pepper to taste

Instructions:

- Toast the bread.

- Spread the mashed avocado on the toast.

- Top with the poached egg and season with salt and pepper.

Greek Yogurt Parfait:

Ingredients:

- 1 cup Greek yogurt

- 1/2 cup mixed berries (e.g., blueberries, strawberries)

- 1 tablespoon honey

- 2 tablespoons chopped nuts (e.g., almonds, walnuts)

Instructions:

- Layer Greek yogurt, mixed berries, honey, and chopped nuts in a glass or bowl.

- Repeat the layers as desired.

Spinach and Mushroom Omelette:

Ingredients:

- 2 large eggs

- 1/2 cup spinach, chopped

- 1/4 cup mushrooms, sliced

- 1/4 cup diced bell peppers

- Salt and pepper to taste

Instructions:

- Whisk the eggs in a bowl and season with salt and pepper.

- Heat a non-stick skillet over medium heat, add a bit of olive oil.

- Sauté the spinach, mushrooms, and bell peppers until tender.

- Pour the beaten eggs over the veggies and cook until set. Fold in half and serve.

Chia Seed Pudding:

Ingredients:

- 2 tablespoons chia seeds

- 1 cup almond milk (or any preferred milk)

- 1/2 teaspoon vanilla extract

- 1 tablespoon honey

- Fresh berries for topping

Instructions:

- Mix chia seeds, almond milk, vanilla extract, and honey in a bowl.

- Refrigerate for at least 2 hours or overnight until it thickens.

- Top with fresh berries before serving.

Banana and Almond Butter Smoothie:

Ingredients:

- 1 ripe banana

- 1 tablespoon almond butter

- 1 cup almond milk (or any preferred milk)

- 1/2 teaspoon cinnamon

- 1 teaspoon honey (optional)

Instructions:

• Blend all ingredients until smooth and creamy.

Quinoa Breakfast Bowl:

Ingredients:

• 1/2 cup cooked quinoa

• 1/4 cup Greek yogurt

• 1/4 cup mixed berries

• 1 tablespoon chopped nuts (e.g., pistachios, almonds)

• 1 teaspoon honey

Instructions:

• In a bowl, layer cooked quinoa, Greek yogurt, mixed berries, nuts, and drizzle with honey.

Sweet Potato Hash:

Ingredients:

• 1 sweet potato, diced

• 1/2 red onion, chopped

• 1/2 bell pepper, diced

• 2 eggs

• Olive oil

• Salt and pepper to taste

Instructions:

• In a skillet, sauté sweet potato, onion, and bell pepper in olive oil until tender.

• Make two wells in the mixture and crack an egg into each.

• Cover and cook until the eggs are done to your liking. Season with salt and pepper.

Turmeric and Ginger Tea:

Ingredients:

- 1 cup hot water

- 1/2 teaspoon turmeric powder

- 1/4 teaspoon grated ginger

- 1 teaspoon honey (optional)

Instructions:

- Mix turmeric powder and grated ginger in hot water.

- Add honey if desired, and stir well.

Mango and Coconut Chia Pudding:

Ingredients:

- 2 tablespoons chia seeds

- 1 cup coconut milk

- 1/2 ripe mango, diced

- 1 tablespoon shredded coconut

- 1 teaspoon honey (optional)

Instructions:

- Mix chia seeds and coconut milk in a bowl.

- Refrigerate for at least 2 hours or until it thickens.

- Top with diced mango, shredded coconut, and honey if desired.

Oatmeal with Berries and Almonds:

Ingredients:

- 1/2 cup rolled oats

- 1 cup almond milk

- 1/4 cup mixed berries (e.g., raspberries, blueberries)

- 1 tablespoon chopped almonds

- 1 teaspoon honey

Instructions:

• Cook oats in almond milk until creamy.

• Top with mixed berries, chopped almonds, and honey.

Smoked Salmon and Avocado Wrap:

Ingredients:

• 1 whole-grain tortilla

• 2 slices smoked salmon

• 1/2 ripe avocado, sliced

• 1 tablespoon Greek yogurt

• Fresh dill (optional)

Instructions:

• Spread Greek yogurt on the tortilla.

• Layer smoked salmon, avocado slices, and fresh dill.

• Roll up and enjoy.

Egg and Veggie Breakfast Burrito:

Ingredients:

• 2 large eggs, scrambled

• 1 whole-grain tortilla

• 1/4 cup bell peppers, diced

• 1/4 cup spinach, chopped

• 1/4 cup black beans, drained and rinsed

• Salsa (optional)

Instructions:

• Cook scrambled eggs, bell peppers, spinach, and black beans in a skillet.

• Warm the tortilla, then fill it with the egg and veggie mixture.

• Add salsa if desired and roll up.

Coconut and Blueberry Pancakes:

Ingredients:

• 1/2 cup coconut flour

• 2 eggs

• 1/2 cup almond milk

• 1/2 teaspoon baking powder

• 1/2 cup blueberries

• 1 tablespoon honey

Instructions:

• In a bowl, whisk together coconut flour, eggs, almond milk, and baking powder.

• Fold in blueberries.

• Cook pancakes on a griddle until golden brown.

• Drizzle with honey before serving.

Green Breakfast Smoothie:

Ingredients:

- 1 cup spinach leaves

- 1/2 ripe banana

- 1/2 cup pineapple chunks

- 1/2 cup almond milk

- 1 tablespoon chia seeds

Instructions:

- Blend all ingredients until smooth.

Coconut and Almond Oat Bars:

Ingredients:

- 1 cup rolled oats

- 1/2 cup almond butter

- 1/4 cup shredded coconut

- 1/4 cup honey

- 1/4 cup chopped almonds

Instructions:

• Mix rolled oats, almond butter, shredded coconut, honey, and chopped almonds in a bowl.

• Press the mixture into a lined baking dish.

• Refrigerate until firm, then cut into bars.

Fruit Salad with Mint and Lime:

Ingredients:

• Assorted fresh fruits (e.g., watermelon, pineapple, strawberries, kiwi)

• Fresh mint leaves

• Juice of 1 lime

• 1 tablespoon honey

Instructions:

• Dice the fruits and combine in a bowl.

• Drizzle with lime juice, honey, and garnish with fresh mint leaves.

Quinoa and Berry Breakfast Bowl:

Ingredients:

• 1/2 cup cooked quinoa

• 1/4 cup mixed berries (e.g., raspberries, blackberries)

• 1 tablespoon chopped nuts (e.g., pecans, walnuts)

• 1 tablespoon honey or maple syrup

Instructions:

• In a bowl, combine cooked quinoa, mixed berries, chopped nuts, and sweeten with honey or maple syrup.

Cinnamon and Apple Overnight Oats:

Ingredients:

- 1/2 cup rolled oats

- 1/2 cup almond milk

- 1/2 apple, diced

- 1/2 teaspoon cinnamon

- 1 teaspoon honey

Instructions:

- Mix rolled oats, almond milk, diced apple, and cinnamon in a jar.

- Refrigerate overnight and drizzle with honey before serving.

Egg and Veggie Breakfast Casserole:

Ingredients:

- 6 eggs, beaten

- 1 cup spinach, chopped

- 1/2 cup cherry tomatoes, halved

- 1/4 cup feta cheese, crumbled

- Salt and pepper to taste

Instructions:

- Preheat the oven to 350°F (175°C).

- Grease a baking dish.

- Mix beaten eggs, spinach, cherry tomatoes, and feta cheese in a bowl.

- Pour the mixture into the baking dish and bake for about 25-30 minutes until set.

Sautéed Asparagus and Poached Eggs:

Ingredients:

- 1 bunch of asparagus

- 2 poached eggs

- Olive oil

- Lemon zest (optional)

• Salt and pepper to taste

Instructions:

• Sauté asparagus spears in olive oil until tender.

• Top with poached eggs, lemon zest, and season with salt and pepper.

LUNCH

Spinach and Quinoa Salad:

Ingredients:

• 1 cup cooked quinoa

• 2 cups fresh spinach leaves

• 1/2 cup cherry tomatoes, halved

• 1/4 cup chickpeas

• 2 tablespoons feta cheese (optional)

• Olive oil and balsamic vinegar for dressing

Instructions:

- Combine quinoa, spinach, cherry tomatoes, and chickpeas in a bowl.

- Top with feta cheese, if desired.

- Drizzle with olive oil and balsamic vinegar for dressing.

Mediterranean Hummus Wrap:

Ingredients:

- 1 whole-grain tortilla

- 2 tablespoons hummus

- 1/4 cup cucumber, thinly sliced

- 1/4 cup bell peppers, thinly sliced

- 1/4 cup cherry tomatoes, halved

- 2 tablespoons feta cheese

Instructions:

- Spread hummus on the tortilla.

• Layer with cucumber, bell peppers, cherry tomatoes, and feta cheese.

• Roll up and enjoy.

Salmon and Quinoa Bowl:

Ingredients:

• 4 oz grilled salmon

• 1 cup cooked quinoa

• 1/2 cup steamed broccoli

• 1/4 cup shredded carrots

• Lemon-Dill dressing (lemon juice, olive oil, fresh dill)

Instructions:

• Place grilled salmon, quinoa, steamed broccoli, and shredded carrots in a bowl.

• Drizzle with Lemon-Dill dressing.

Veggie and Lentil Soup:

Ingredients:

• 1 cup green lentils

• 4 cups vegetable broth

• 1 cup mixed vegetables (e.g., carrots, celery, onions)

• 2 cloves garlic, minced

• 1 teaspoon turmeric

• Salt and pepper to taste

Instructions:

• Rinse lentils and combine them with vegetable broth, mixed vegetables, garlic, turmeric, salt, and pepper in a large pot.

• Bring to a boil, then simmer until lentils and vegetables are tender.

Greek Quinoa Salad:

Ingredients:

• 1 cup cooked quinoa

• 1/2 cup diced cucumber

• 1/2 cup diced tomatoes

• 1/4 cup Kalamata olives, pitted and sliced

• 1/4 cup crumbled feta cheese

• Olive oil and lemon juice for dressing

Instructions:

• Combine quinoa, cucumber, tomatoes, Kalamata olives, and feta cheese in a bowl.

• Drizzle with olive oil and lemon juice for dressing.

Roasted Vegetable Wrap:

Ingredients:

• 1 whole-grain tortilla

- 1/2 cup roasted vegetables (e.g., zucchini, bell peppers, eggplant)

- 2 tablespoons hummus

- Fresh basil leaves

Instructions:

- Spread hummus on the tortilla.

- Layer with roasted vegetables and fresh basil leaves.

- Roll up and enjoy.

Lemon-Dill Salmon Salad:

Ingredients:

- 4 oz grilled or baked salmon

- 2 cups mixed greens

- 1/4 cup sliced cucumber

- 1/4 cup cherry tomatoes, halved

• Lemon-Dill dressing (lemon juice, olive oil, fresh dill)

Instructions:

• Place grilled salmon on a bed of mixed greens.

• Top with sliced cucumber and cherry tomatoes.

• Drizzle with Lemon-Dill dressing.

Sweet Potato and Chickpea Curry:

Ingredients:

• 1 large sweet potato, diced

• 1 can chickpeas, drained and rinsed

• 1 onion, chopped

• 2 cloves garlic, minced

• 1 can coconut milk

• 2 tablespoons curry powder

• Salt and pepper to taste

Instructions:

• Sauté onions and garlic in a large pot until fragrant.

• Add sweet potato, chickpeas, coconut milk, curry powder, salt, and pepper.

• Simmer until sweet potatoes are tender.

Caprese Salad with Quinoa:

Ingredients:

• 1 cup cooked quinoa

• 1 cup cherry tomatoes, halved

• 1/2 cup fresh mozzarella balls

• Fresh basil leaves

• Balsamic glaze for drizzling

Instructions:

• Combine quinoa, cherry tomatoes, fresh mozzarella, and basil leaves in a bowl.

• Drizzle with balsamic glaze.

Turkey and Avocado Wrap:

Ingredients:

• 1 whole-grain tortilla

• 2 slices roasted turkey breast

• 1/2 avocado, sliced

• 1/4 cup mixed greens

• Dijon mustard (optional)

Instructions:

• Layer turkey, avocado slices, mixed greens, and Dijon mustard (if desired) on the tortilla.

• Roll up and enjoy.

Cauliflower and Leek Soup:

Ingredients:

- 1 head cauliflower, chopped

- 2 leeks, chopped

- 1 clove garlic, minced

- 4 cups vegetable broth

- Olive oil

- Salt and pepper to taste

Instructions:

- Sauté leeks and garlic in olive oil until softened.

- Add cauliflower and vegetable broth.

- Simmer until cauliflower is tender, then blend until smooth.

Quinoa and Black Bean Salad:

Ingredients:

- 1 cup cooked quinoa

- 1 can black beans, drained and rinsed

- 1/2 cup corn kernels (fresh or frozen)

- 1/4 cup red bell pepper, diced

- 2 tablespoons fresh cilantro, chopped

- Lime vinaigrette (lime juice, olive oil, cumin)

Instructions:

- Mix quinoa, black beans, corn, red bell pepper, and cilantro in a bowl.

- Drizzle with lime vinaigrette.

Chicken and Vegetable Stir-Fry:

Ingredients:

- 4 oz cooked chicken breast, sliced

- 1 cup mixed vegetables (e.g., broccoli, bell peppers, snap peas)

- 2 cloves garlic, minced

- Low-sodium soy sauce

• Sesame oil

• Ginger (fresh or powdered)

Instructions:

• Stir-fry mixed vegetables and garlic in sesame oil until tender.

• Add sliced chicken, ginger, and a splash of low-sodium soy sauce. Cook until heated through.

Eggplant and Tomato Salad:

Ingredients:

• 1 eggplant, sliced and grilled

• 1 cup cherry tomatoes, halved

• 1/4 cup fresh basil leaves

• Balsamic glaze for drizzling

Instructions:

• Arrange grilled eggplant, cherry tomatoes, and fresh basil on a plate.

• Drizzle with balsamic glaze.

Tuna and White Bean Salad:

Ingredients:

• 1 can white beans, drained and rinsed

• 1 can tuna, drained

• 1/4 cup red onion, finely chopped

• 1/4 cup fresh parsley, chopped

• Olive oil and lemon juice for dressing

Instructions:

• Combine white beans, tuna, red onion, and fresh parsley in a bowl.

• Drizzle with olive oil and lemon juice for dressing.

Shrimp and Asparagus Stir-Fry:

Ingredients:

• 4 oz shrimp, peeled and deveined

• 1 bunch asparagus, trimmed and cut into pieces

• 2 cloves garlic, minced

• Low-sodium soy sauce

• Sesame oil

• Red pepper flakes (optional)

Instructions:

• Stir-fry asparagus and garlic in sesame oil until tender.

• Add shrimp and a splash of low-sodium soy sauce. Cook until shrimp turn pink.

• Sprinkle with red pepper flakes if desired.

Butternut Squash and Carrot Soup:

Ingredients:

• 2 cups butternut squash, diced

• 1 cup carrots, sliced

• 1 onion, chopped

• 4 cups vegetable broth

• 1/2 teaspoon ground ginger

• Salt and pepper to taste

Instructions:

• Sauté onions in a large pot until translucent.

• Add butternut squash, carrots, vegetable broth, ginger, salt, and pepper.

• Simmer until vegetables are tender, then blend until smooth.

Tofu and Vegetable Stir-Fry:

Ingredients:

• 1/2 block firm tofu, cubed

• 1 cup mixed vegetables (e.g., broccoli, bell peppers, snap peas)

• 2 cloves garlic, minced

• Low-sodium soy sauce

• Sesame oil

• Sesame seeds (optional)

Instructions:

• Stir-fry mixed vegetables and garlic in sesame oil until tender.

• Add cubed tofu and a splash of low-sodium soy sauce. Cook until heated through.

• Garnish with sesame seeds if desired.

Chickpea and Cucumber Salad:

Ingredients:

- 1 can chickpeas, drained and rinsed

- 1/2 cucumber, diced

- 1/4 cup red onion, finely chopped

- 2 tablespoons fresh mint leaves, chopped

- Lemon vinaigrette (lemon juice, olive oil, Dijon mustard)

Instructions:

- Combine chickpeas, cucumber, red onion, and fresh mint in a bowl.

- Drizzle with lemon vinaigrette.

Sesame Ginger Tofu Bowl:

Ingredients:

- 1/2 block firm tofu, cubed and pan-fried

- 1 cup cooked brown rice

- 1 cup steamed broccoli

- 1/4 cup shredded carrots

- Sesame ginger sauce (soy sauce, sesame oil, ginger, garlic)

- Sesame seeds for garnish

Instructions:

- Assemble cooked tofu, brown rice, steamed broccoli, and shredded carrots in a bowl.

- Drizzle with sesame ginger sauce and garnish with sesame seeds.

DINNER

Lemon Garlic Roasted Chicken:

Ingredients:

- 4 boneless, skinless chicken breasts

- 2 lemons (zest and juice)

- 4 cloves garlic, minced

- Fresh rosemary sprigs

• Olive oil

• Salt and pepper to taste

Instructions:

• Preheat the oven to 375°F (190°C).

• In a bowl, mix lemon zest, lemon juice, minced garlic, and olive oil.

• Place chicken breasts in a baking dish, pour the lemon-garlic mixture over them, and season with salt and pepper.

• Add fresh rosemary sprigs on top.

• Roast in the oven for about 25-30 minutes or until the chicken is cooked through.

Baked Salmon with Dill Sauce:

Ingredients:

• 4 salmon fillets

• 2 tablespoons fresh dill, chopped

- 2 cloves garlic, minced

- 1 lemon, sliced

- Olive oil

- Salt and pepper to taste

Instructions:

- Preheat the oven to 375°F (190°C).

- Place salmon fillets in a baking dish.

- Mix chopped dill, minced garlic, olive oil, salt, and pepper in a bowl.

- Pour the dill mixture over the salmon and top with lemon slices.

- Bake for about 15-20 minutes or until the salmon flakes easily.

Mushroom and Spinach Stuffed Bell Peppers:

Ingredients:

- 4 bell peppers, halved and seeds removed

- 1 cup mushrooms, chopped

- 2 cups spinach leaves

- 1 cup cooked quinoa

- 1/4 cup grated Parmesan cheese

- Olive oil

- Salt and pepper to taste

Instructions:

- Preheat the oven to 375°F (190°C).

- Lightly brush the outside of bell pepper halves with olive oil and place them in a baking dish.

- Sauté mushrooms and spinach in olive oil until wilted.

- Mix the sautéed vegetables with cooked quinoa, Parmesan cheese, salt, and pepper.

- Stuff the bell pepper halves with the quinoa mixture.

• Bake for about 20-25 minutes or until peppers are tender.

Grilled Vegetable and Chickpea Salad:

Ingredients:

• Assorted vegetables (e.g., zucchini, eggplant, bell peppers)

• 1 can chickpeas, drained and rinsed

• Fresh basil leaves

• Balsamic vinaigrette (balsamic vinegar, olive oil, Dijon mustard)

• Salt and pepper to taste

Instructions:

• Grill the assorted vegetables until tender.

• Combine grilled vegetables, chickpeas, fresh basil leaves, and a drizzle of balsamic vinaigrette in a bowl.

• Season with salt and pepper.

Turkey and Vegetable Stir-Fry:

Ingredients:

• 1 lb ground turkey

• 2 cups mixed vegetables (e.g., broccoli, bell peppers, snap peas)

• 2 cloves garlic, minced

• Low-sodium soy sauce

• Sesame oil

• Ginger (fresh or powdered)

Instructions:

• In a large skillet, brown ground turkey until cooked through.

• Remove turkey from the skillet and set aside.

• Stir-fry mixed vegetables and garlic in sesame oil until tender.

• Add cooked turkey back to the skillet, along with a splash of low-sodium soy sauce and ginger. Cook until heated through.

Baked Cod with Tomato and Olive Tapenade:

Ingredients:

• 4 cod fillets

• 1 cup cherry tomatoes, halved

• 1/4 cup Kalamata olives, pitted and sliced

• 2 cloves garlic, minced

• Olive oil

• Fresh basil leaves

• Salt and pepper to taste

Instructions:

- Preheat the oven to 375°F (190°C).

- Place cod fillets in a baking dish.

- Mix cherry tomatoes, Kalamata olives, minced garlic, olive oil, salt, and pepper in a bowl.

- Spoon the tomato and olive mixture over the cod.

- Bake for about 15-20 minutes or until the cod flakes easily.

- Garnish with fresh basil leaves.

Stuffed Portobello Mushrooms:

Ingredients:

- 4 large Portobello mushrooms

- 1 cup quinoa, cooked

- 1 cup spinach, chopped

- 1/4 cup feta cheese

- Olive oil

• Balsamic glaze

• Salt and pepper to taste

Instructions:

• Preheat the oven to 375°F (190°C).

• Remove the stems from Portobello mushrooms and brush with olive oil.

• In a bowl, mix cooked quinoa, chopped spinach, feta cheese, salt, and pepper.

• Stuff the mushrooms with the quinoa mixture.

• Bake for about 20-25 minutes or until mushrooms are tender.

• Drizzle with balsamic glaze before serving.

Lentil and Vegetable Curry:

Ingredients:

• 1 cup green or brown lentils

• 2 cups vegetable broth

• Assorted vegetables (e.g., cauliflower, carrots, bell peppers)

• 1 can coconut milk

• Curry paste or powder

• Salt and pepper to taste

Instructions:

• Rinse lentils and combine them with vegetable broth, assorted vegetables, coconut milk, curry paste or powder, salt, and pepper in a large pot.

• Simmer until lentils and vegetables are tender.

Shrimp and Zucchini Noodles:

Ingredients:

• 8 oz shrimp, peeled and deveined

• 2 large zucchinis, spiralized into noodles

• 2 cloves garlic, minced

• Olive oil

• Lemon zest and juice

• Fresh basil leaves

• Salt and pepper to taste

Instructions:

• Sauté shrimp and minced garlic in olive oil until shrimp turn pink.

• Add zucchini noodles and cook until tender.

• Toss with lemon zest, lemon juice, fresh basil leaves, salt, and pepper.

Chickpea and Sweet Potato Curry:

Ingredients:

• 2 cups diced sweet potatoes

• 1 can chickpeas, drained and rinsed

- 1 onion, chopped

- 2 cloves garlic, minced

- 1 can coconut milk

- Curry paste or powder

- Olive oil

- Salt and pepper to taste

Instructions:

- Sauté onions and garlic in olive oil until translucent.

- Add diced sweet potatoes, chickpeas, coconut milk, curry paste or powder, salt, and pepper.

- Simmer until sweet potatoes are tender.

Lemon Herb Grilled Chicken:

Ingredients:

- 4 boneless, skinless chicken breasts

• 2 lemons (zest and juice)

• 2 tablespoons fresh herbs (e.g., rosemary, thyme, parsley), chopped

• Olive oil

• Salt and pepper to taste

Instructions:

• Preheat the grill to medium-high heat.

• In a bowl, mix lemon zest, lemon juice, chopped herbs, olive oil, salt, and pepper.

• Brush the chicken breasts with the lemon herb mixture.

• Grill the chicken for about 6-8 minutes per side or until cooked through.

Cauliflower Rice Stir-Fry with Tofu:

Ingredients:

• 1/2 block firm tofu, cubed

- 1 head cauliflower, grated into "rice"

- 2 cups mixed vegetables (e.g., broccoli, snap peas, bell peppers)

- Low-sodium soy sauce

- Sesame oil

- Garlic powder

- Ginger (fresh or powdered)

Instructions:

- Sauté cubed tofu in sesame oil until lightly browned.

- Add mixed vegetables, cauliflower rice, low-sodium soy sauce, garlic powder, and ginger. Cook until heated through.

Baked Eggplant Parmesan:

Ingredients:

- 2 large eggplants, sliced

- 1 cup whole wheat breadcrumbs

- 1/4 cup grated Parmesan cheese

- 2 cups marinara sauce

- 1 cup mozzarella cheese, shredded

- Fresh basil leaves

- Olive oil

- Salt and pepper to taste

Instructions:

- Preheat the oven to 375°F (190°C).

- Brush eggplant slices with olive oil and bake for about 20-25 minutes until tender.

- In a bowl, mix breadcrumbs, grated Parmesan, salt, and pepper.

- In a baking dish, layer baked eggplant, marinara sauce, breadcrumb mixture, and mozzarella cheese.

- Bake for about 20-25 minutes or until cheese is melted and bubbly.

• Garnish with fresh basil leaves before serving.

75

Teriyaki Salmon with Broccoli:

Ingredients:

• 4 salmon fillets

• 2 cups broccoli florets

• Teriyaki sauce (store-bought or homemade)

• Olive oil

• Sesame seeds (optional)

• Salt and pepper to taste

Instructions:

• Preheat the oven to 375°F (190°C).

• Place salmon fillets on a baking sheet.

• Toss broccoli florets with olive oil, salt, and pepper, and spread them on the same baking sheet.

• Brush salmon with teriyaki sauce and sprinkle with sesame seeds (if desired).

• Bake for about 15-20 minutes or until salmon flakes easily.

Cabbage and White Bean Soup:

Ingredients:

• 1 small cabbage, shredded

• 1 can white beans, drained and rinsed

• 1 onion, chopped

• 2 cloves garlic, minced

• 4 cups vegetable broth

• Olive oil

• Paprika

• Salt and pepper to taste

Instructions:

• Sauté onions and garlic in olive oil until translucent.

• Add shredded cabbage, white beans, vegetable broth, paprika, salt, and pepper.

• Simmer until cabbage is tender.

Tofu and Vegetable Curry:

Ingredients:

• 1/2 block firm tofu, cubed

• 2 cups mixed vegetables (e.g., bell peppers, zucchini, carrots)

• 2 cloves garlic, minced

• Coconut milk

• Red curry paste

• Lime juice

• Salt and pepper to taste

Instructions:

• Sauté cubed tofu and minced garlic in a large skillet until lightly browned.

• Add mixed vegetables and sauté until tender.

• Stir in coconut milk, red curry paste, lime juice, salt, and pepper. Simmer until heated through.

Mediterranean Stuffed Peppers:

Ingredients:

• 4 bell peppers, halved and seeds removed

• 1 cup cooked quinoa

• 1/2 cup cherry tomatoes, halved

• 1/4 cup Kalamata olives, pitted and sliced

• 1/4 cup crumbled feta cheese

• Olive oil

• Fresh basil leaves

• Salt and pepper to taste

Instructions:

• Preheat the oven to 375°F (190°C).

• Lightly brush the outside of bell pepper halves with olive oil and place them in a baking dish.

• Mix cooked quinoa, cherry tomatoes, Kalamata olives, crumbled feta cheese, salt, and pepper in a bowl.

• Stuff the bell pepper halves with the quinoa mixture.

• Bake for about 20-25 minutes or until peppers are tender.

• Garnish with fresh basil leaves before serving.

Black Bean and Vegetable Stir-Fry:

Ingredients:

• 1 can black beans, drained and rinsed

- 2 cups mixed vegetables (e.g., broccoli, bell peppers, snap peas)

- 2 cloves garlic, minced

- Low-sodium soy sauce

- Sesame oil

- Ginger (fresh or powdered)

Instructions:

- Stir-fry mixed vegetables and minced garlic in sesame oil until tender.

- Add black beans, a splash of low-sodium soy sauce, and ginger. Cook until heated through.

Lemon Herb Roasted Vegetables:

Ingredients:

- Assorted vegetables (e.g., carrots, potatoes, Brussels sprouts)

• 2 tablespoons fresh herbs (e.g., rosemary, thyme, parsley), chopped

• 2 cloves garlic, minced

• Olive oil

• Lemon zest and juice

• Salt and pepper to taste

Instructions:

• Preheat the oven to 375°F (190°C).

• Toss assorted vegetables with olive oil, fresh herbs, minced garlic, lemon zest, lemon juice, salt, and pepper.

• Roast in the oven for about 30-40 minutes or until vegetables are tender and slightly caramelized.

Vegan Lentil Shepherd's Pie:

Ingredients:

• 2 cups cooked green or brown lentils

- 2 cups mixed vegetables (e.g., carrots, peas, corn)

- 1 onion, chopped

- 2 cloves garlic, minced

- Mashed potatoes (made with almond milk and vegan butter)

- Olive oil

- Salt and pepper to taste

Instructions:

- Sauté onions and garlic in olive oil until translucent.

- Add cooked lentils, mixed vegetables, salt, and pepper. Cook until heated through.

- Transfer the lentil and vegetable mixture to a baking dish.

- Top with mashed potatoes and bake for about 20-25 minutes or until the top is golden brown.

Avocado and Tomato Bruschetta:

Ingredients:

• Whole-grain baguette slices

• Ripe avocados, mashed

• Cherry tomatoes, diced

• Fresh basil leaves, chopped

• Olive oil

• Balsamic vinegar

• Salt and pepper to taste

Instructions:

• Toast whole-grain baguette slices.

• Spread mashed avocado on each slice.

• Top with diced cherry tomatoes and chopped fresh basil.

• Drizzle with olive oil and balsamic vinegar. Season with salt and pepper.

Greek Yogurt with Berries and Honey:

Ingredients:

• Greek yogurt

• Fresh mixed berries (e.g., strawberries, blueberries, raspberries)

• Honey

Instructions:

• Spoon Greek yogurt into a bowl.

• Top with fresh mixed berries.

• Drizzle with honey.

Hummus and Veggie Platter:

Ingredients:

• Hummus

• Assorted vegetable sticks (e.g., carrots, cucumbers, bell peppers)

Instructions:

• Arrange a variety of vegetable sticks on a platter.

• Serve with hummus for dipping.

Trail Mix:

Ingredients:

• Mixed nuts (e.g., almonds, walnuts, cashews)

• Dried fruits (e.g., raisins, apricots, cranberries)

• Dark chocolate chips or chunks

Instructions:

• Mix the nuts, dried fruits, and dark chocolate in a bowl.

• Portion into small snack-sized bags.

Cottage Cheese with Pineapple:

Ingredients:

• Low-fat cottage cheese

• Fresh pineapple chunks

Instructions:

• Spoon low-fat cottage cheese into a bowl.

• Top with fresh pineapple chunks.

Almond and Date Energy Balls:

Ingredients:

• 1 cup almonds

• 1 cup pitted dates

• Unsweetened shredded coconut (optional)

Instructions:

- Blend almonds and dates in a food processor until well combined.

- Roll the mixture into bite-sized balls.

- Optionally, roll in unsweetened shredded coconut.

Cucumber and Smoked Salmon Bites:

Ingredients:

- Cucumber slices

- Smoked salmon

- Cream cheese (optional)

Instructions:

- Lay cucumber slices on a plate.

- Top each cucumber slice with smoked salmon and a small dollop of cream cheese if desired.

Cherry Tomatoes with Fresh Basil:

Ingredients:

• Cherry tomatoes

• Fresh basil leaves

• Balsamic glaze

• Fresh mozzarella balls (optional)

Instructions:

• Skewer cherry tomatoes and fresh basil leaves alternately.

• Drizzle with balsamic glaze.

• Optionally, add fresh mozzarella balls to the skewers.

Walnut and Berry Parfait:

Ingredients:

• Greek yogurt

• Chopped walnuts

• Mixed berries (e.g., strawberries, blueberries, raspberries)

• Honey

Instructions:

• Layer Greek yogurt, chopped walnuts, and mixed berries in a glass or bowl.

• Drizzle with honey.

Chia Pudding with Almonds and Berries:

Ingredients:

• 2 tablespoons chia seeds

• 1 cup almond milk

• Sliced almonds

• Mixed berries

• Honey

Instructions:

• Mix chia seeds and almond milk in a jar. Refrigerate for a few hours or overnight until it thickens.

• Top with sliced almonds, mixed berries, and a drizzle of honey.

Apple Slices with Almond Butter:

Ingredients:

• Apple slices

• Almond butter

Instructions:

• Spread almond butter on apple slices.

Sliced Cucumber with Tzatziki:

Ingredients:

• Cucumber slices

• Tzatziki sauce

Instructions:

• Serve cucumber slices with a side of tzatziki sauce for dipping.

Baked Sweet Potato Fries:

Ingredients:

• Sweet potatoes, cut into fries

• Olive oil

• Paprika

• Salt and pepper to taste

Instructions:

• Toss sweet potato fries with olive oil, paprika, salt, and pepper.

• Bake in a preheated oven at 425°F (220°C) for about 20-25 minutes or until crispy.

Mango and Papaya Salsa with Jicama:

Ingredients:

• Mango, diced

• Papaya, diced

• Jicama sticks

• Fresh lime juice

• Fresh cilantro leaves

• Jalapeño pepper (optional, for heat)

• Salt and pepper to taste

Instructions:

• Mix diced mango, papaya, lime juice, fresh cilantro, and jalapeño pepper (if using) in a bowl.

• Serve with jicama sticks for dipping.

Yogurt and Cinnamon Apple Slices:

Ingredients:

• Greek yogurt

• Apple slices

• Ground cinnamon

• Honey (optional)

Instructions:

• Dip apple slices in Greek yogurt.

• Sprinkle with ground cinnamon and drizzle with honey if desired.

Mixed Berry Parfait:

• Ingredients:

• Greek yogurt

• Mixed berries (e.g., strawberries, blueberries, raspberries)

• Honey

Instructions:

• Layer Greek yogurt and mixed berries in a glass.

• Drizzle with honey.

Dark Chocolate-Dipped Strawberries:

Ingredients:

• Fresh strawberries

• Dark chocolate chips

Instructions:

• Melt dark chocolate chips in a microwave or on the stove.

• Dip fresh strawberries into the melted chocolate and place them on a parchment paper-lined tray to cool and harden.

Baked Apples with Cinnamon and Walnuts:

Ingredients:

• Apples (e.g., Granny Smith)

• Cinnamon

• Chopped walnuts

• Honey (optional)

Instructions:

• Core and slice apples.

• Place apple slices in a baking dish, sprinkle with cinnamon, and top with chopped walnuts.

• Optionally, drizzle with honey.

• Bake in a preheated oven at 350°F (175°C) for about 20-25 minutes or until apples are tender.

Chia Seed Pudding with Berries:

Ingredients:

• 3 tablespoons chia seeds

• 1 cup almond milk

• Mixed berries (e.g., strawberries, blueberries, raspberries)

• Honey (optional)

Instructions:

• Mix chia seeds and almond milk in a jar. Refrigerate for a few hours or overnight until it thickens.

• Top with mixed berries and a drizzle of honey.

Frozen Banana Bites:

Ingredients:

• Ripe bananas, sliced into rounds

• Almond butter

• Dark chocolate chips

Instructions:

• Spread almond butter between banana rounds to create sandwiches.

• Dip banana sandwiches into melted dark chocolate and place them on a parchment paper-lined tray.

• Freeze until chocolate hardens.

Yogurt and Berry Popsicles:

Ingredients:

• Greek yogurt

• Mixed berries (e.g., strawberries, blueberries, raspberries)

• Honey (optional)

Instructions:

• Mix Greek yogurt, mixed berries, and honey (if desired) in a blender until smooth.

• Pour the mixture into popsicle molds and freeze until solid.

Cinnamon Roasted Almonds:

Ingredients:

• Raw almonds

• Ground cinnamon

• Honey

Instructions:

• Toss raw almonds with ground cinnamon and a drizzle of honey.

• Roast in a preheated oven at 350°F (175°C) for about 10-15 minutes or until fragrant and lightly toasted.

Coconut Date Balls:

Ingredients:

• Medjool dates, pitted

• Unsweetened shredded coconut

• Almonds

Instructions:

• Blend pitted dates, shredded coconut, and almonds in a food processor until the mixture comes together.

• Roll into bite-sized balls.

Baked Pears with Honey and Cinnamon:

Ingredients:

• Ripe pears, halved and cored

• Honey

• Ground cinnamon

• Chopped pecans

Instructions:

- Place pear halves in a baking dish.

- Drizzle with honey, sprinkle with ground cinnamon, and top with chopped pecans.

- Bake in a preheated oven at 350°F (175°C) for about 20-25 minutes or until pears are tender.

Frozen Blueberry Yogurt Bark:

Ingredients:

- Greek yogurt

- Frozen blueberries

- Honey (optional)

Instructions:

- Mix Greek yogurt and frozen blueberries.

- Spread the mixture on a parchment paper-lined tray.

- Drizzle with honey if desired.

• Freeze until solid, then break into pieces.

Chocolate Avocado Mousse:

Ingredients:

• Ripe avocados

• Unsweetened cocoa powder

• Honey

Instructions:

• Blend ripe avocados, unsweetened cocoa powder, and honey in a food processor until smooth.

• Chill in the refrigerator before serving.

• Oatmeal Banana Cookies:

Ingredients:

• Ripe bananas, mashed

• Rolled oats

• Cinnamon

• Dark chocolate chips (optional)

Instructions:

• Mix mashed bananas, rolled oats, cinnamon, and dark chocolate chips (if using).

• Drop spoonfuls of the mixture onto a baking sheet.

• Bake in a preheated oven at 350°F (175°C) for about 15-20 minutes or until cookies are set.

Pumpkin Spice Energy Bites:

Ingredients:

• Rolled oats

• Pumpkin puree

• Ground cinnamon

• Chopped pecans

• Honey

Instructions:

• Mix rolled oats, pumpkin puree, ground cinnamon, chopped pecans, and honey in a bowl.

• Roll into bite-sized balls.

Cherry Almond Yogurt Bowl:

Ingredients:

• Greek yogurt

• Fresh or frozen cherries

• Sliced almonds

• Honey (optional)

Instructions:

• Layer Greek yogurt, cherries, sliced almonds, and a drizzle of honey if desired.

Raspberry and Mint Sorbet:

Ingredients:

• Frozen raspberries

• Fresh mint leaves

• Honey (optional)

Instructions:

• Blend frozen raspberries, fresh mint leaves, and honey (if desired) in a blender until smooth.

• Freeze until the mixture reaches a sorbet-like consistency.

CONCLUSION

"Living Well with Vagus Nerve: A Cookbook" offers a holistic approach to enhancing your well-being through mindful eating practices and stress reduction techniques that support the health of your vagus nerve. The cookbook provides a diverse range of recipes, from breakfast to dinner and snacks to desserts, all designed to nourish both your body and your vagus nerve. By incorporating these recipes into your daily life, you can promote relaxation, better digestion, reduced inflammation, and improved overall health.

Remember that a balanced diet rich in whole foods, particularly those that align with the Vagus Nerve Diet, can have a profound impact on your physical and mental well-being. Pairing these recipes with mindfulness in eating and stress reduction techniques can help you harness the power of your vagus nerve for a happier and healthier life.

So, embark on this culinary journey, explore the delicious and nutritious recipes, and embrace a lifestyle that prioritizes the care and well-being of your vagus nerve. In doing so, you'll discover the many benefits of harmonizing your mind, body, and the intricate workings of your nervous system, ultimately living well with your vagus nerve as your trusted guide.